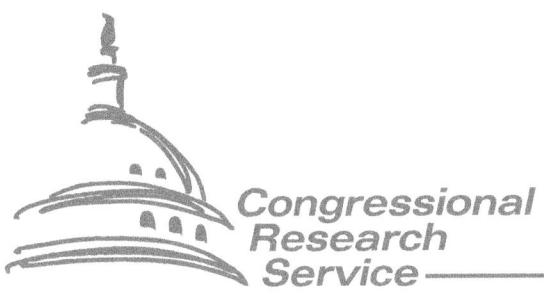

Military Medical Care: Questions and Answers

Don J. Jansen
Analyst in Defense Health Care Policy

Katherine Blakeley
Analyst in Foreign Affairs

October 4, 2012

Congressional Research Service
7-5700
www.crs.gov
RL33537

CRS Report for Congress
Prepared for Members and Committees of Congress

Summary

The primary objective of the military health system, which includes the Defense Department's hospitals, clinics, and medical personnel, is to maintain the health of military personnel so they can carry out their military missions and to be prepared to deliver health care during wartime. The military health system also covers dependents of active duty personnel, military retirees and their dependents, including some members of the reserve components. The military health system provides health care services through either Department of Defense (DOD) medical facilities, known as "military treatment facilities" or "MTFs" as space is available, or through private health care providers. The military health system currently includes some 56 hospitals and 365 clinics serving 9.7 million beneficiaries. It operates worldwide and employs some 58,369 civilians and 86,007 military personnel.

Since 1966, civilian care to millions of dependents and retirees (and retirees' dependents) has been provided through a program still known in law as the Civilian Health and Medical Program of the Uniformed Services (CHAMPUS), but more commonly known as TRICARE. TRICARE has four main benefit plans: a health maintenance organization option (TRICARE Prime), a preferred provider option (TRICARE Extra), a fee-for-service option (TRICARE Standard), and a Medicare wrap-around option (TRICARE for Life) for Medicare-eligible retirees. Other TRICARE plans include TRICARE Young Adult, TRICARE Reserve Select and TRICARE Retired Reserve. TRICARE also includes a pharmacy program and optional dental plans. Options available to beneficiaries vary by the beneficiary's duty status and location.

This report answers several frequently asked questions about military health care, including

- How is the military health system structured?
- What is TRICARE?
- What are the different TRICARE plans and who is eligible?
- What are the costs of military health care to beneficiaries?
- What is the relationship of TRICARE to Medicare?
- How does the Affordable Care Act affect TRICARE?
- What are the long-term trends in defense health care costs?
- What is the Medicare Eligible Retiree Health Care fund, which funds TRICARE for Life?

The Government Accountability Office (GAO) and the Congressional Budget Office (CBO) have also published important studies on the organization, coordination and costs of the military health system, as well as its effectiveness addressing particular health challenges. The Office of the Assistant Secretary of Defense for Health Affairs Home Page, available at http://www.health.mil/, may also be of interest for additional information on the military health system.

Contents

Background 1
Questions and Answers 1
   1. How is the Military Health System Structured? 1
      Administrative Structure 1
      Potential Consolidation 3
      Medical Personnel and Facilities 3
      TRICARE Organization 3
   2. What is the Unified Medical Budget? 4
   3. What is the Medicare Eligible Retiree Health Care Fund (MERHCF)? 6
   4. What is TRICARE? 6
   5. What are the Different TRICARE Plans? 7
      TRICARE Prime 7
      TRICARE Standard 7
      TRICARE Extra 7
      TRICARE Reserve Select 8
      TRICARE Retired Reserve 8
      TRICARE Young Adult 8
      TRICARE for Life 9
   6. How Much Does Military Health Care Cost Beneficiaries? 9
   7. What Is the DOD Pharmacy Benefit? 13
   8. Who Is Eligible to Receive Care? 13
   9. How Are Priorities for Care in Military Medical Facilities Assigned? 14
   10. What are the Long-Term Trends in Defense Health Costs? 15
   11. How Does the Patient Protection and Affordable Care Act Affect TRICARE? 17
   12. How Are Private Health Care Providers Paid? 17
   13. What Is the Relationship of DOD Health Care to Medicare? 18
      TRICARE and Medicare Payments to Providers and the Sustainable Growth Rate 18
      Medicare and TRICARE for Life 18
   14. What Medical Benefits are Available to Reservists? 19
   15. Have Military Personnel Been Promised Free Medical Care for Life? 20
   16. What is the Congressionally Directed Medical Research Program? 20
   17. Other Frequently Asked Questions 22
      Does TRICARE Cover Abortion? 22
      Does DOD Use Animals in Medical Research or Training? 22

Figures

Figure 1. Organization of Health Care Services Provided by DOD 2
Figure 2. FY2013 Unified Medical Budget Request ($billions) 5
Figure 3. Military Health System Eligible Beneficiaries (millions) 14

Tables

Table 1. Selected TRICARE Fees for Active Duty Personnel, Eligible Reservists, and Dependents 9
Table 2. Selected TRICARE Fees for Retirees Under Age 65 and Their Dependents 10
Table 3. Selected TRICARE Fees for Reserve Select and TRICARE Retired Reserve 11
Table 4. Selected TRICARE Fees for TRICARE Young Adult 11
Table 5. TRICARE for Life Fees and Payment Structure 12
Table 6. Appropriation Levels by Fiscal Year(FY) for Selected CDMR Programs, FY2007–FY2012 21

Contacts

Author Contact Information 22

Background

Since 1966, civilian care to millions of dependents and retirees (and retirees' dependents) has been provided through a program still known in law as the Civilian Health and Medical Program of the Uniformed Services (CHAMPUS), but more commonly known as TRICARE. TRICARE has four main benefit plans: a health maintenance organization option (TRICARE Prime), a preferred provider option (TRICARE Extra), a fee-for-service option (TRICARE Standard), and a Medicare wrap-around option (TRICARE for Life) for Medicare-eligible retirees. Other TRICARE plans include TRICARE Young Adult, TRICARE Reserve Select and TRICARE Retired Reserve. TRICARE also includes a pharmacy program and optional dental plans. Options available to beneficiaries vary by the beneficiary's duty status and location.

The Government Accountability Office (GAO) and the Congressional Budget Office (CBO) have also published important studies on the organization, coordination and costs of the military health system, as well as its effectiveness addressing particular health challenges. The Office of the Assistant Secretary of Defense for Health Affairs Home Page, available at http://www.health.mil/, may also be of interest for additional information on the military health system.

Questions and Answers

1. How is the Military Health System Structured?

Administrative Structure

The military health system consists of (1) the Defense Health Program (DHP) which is centrally directed by the Office of the Secretary of Defense and executed by the military departments, and (2) medical resources under the direction of the combatant or support command within the military departments. For DOD, the Assistant Secretary of Defense for Health Affairs (ASD(HA)) controls non-deployable medical resources, facilities and personnel. The ASD(HA) reports to the Under Secretary of Defense for Personnel and Readiness who reports to the Deputy Secretary of Defense. The following all currently report to the ASD/HA:

- Deputy Assistant Secretary of Defense for Clinical and Program Policy
- Deputy Assistant Secretary of Defense for Force Health Protection and Readiness
- Deputy Assistant Secretary of Defense for Health Budget and Financial Policy
- Deputy Director TRICARE Management Activity
- Chief Information Officer for Health
- Director, Strategy and Development
- Director, Communication and Media Relations
- Director, Defense Center of Excellence for Psychological Health and Traumatic Brain Injury
- President, Uniformed Services University of the Health Sciences

Other elements within the Office of the Secretary of Defense, such as the Office of the Director for Program Analysis and Evaluation and the Office of the Under Secretary of Defense (Comptroller), are also responsible for various aspects of the military health system.

Figure 1. Organization of Health Care Services Provided by DOD

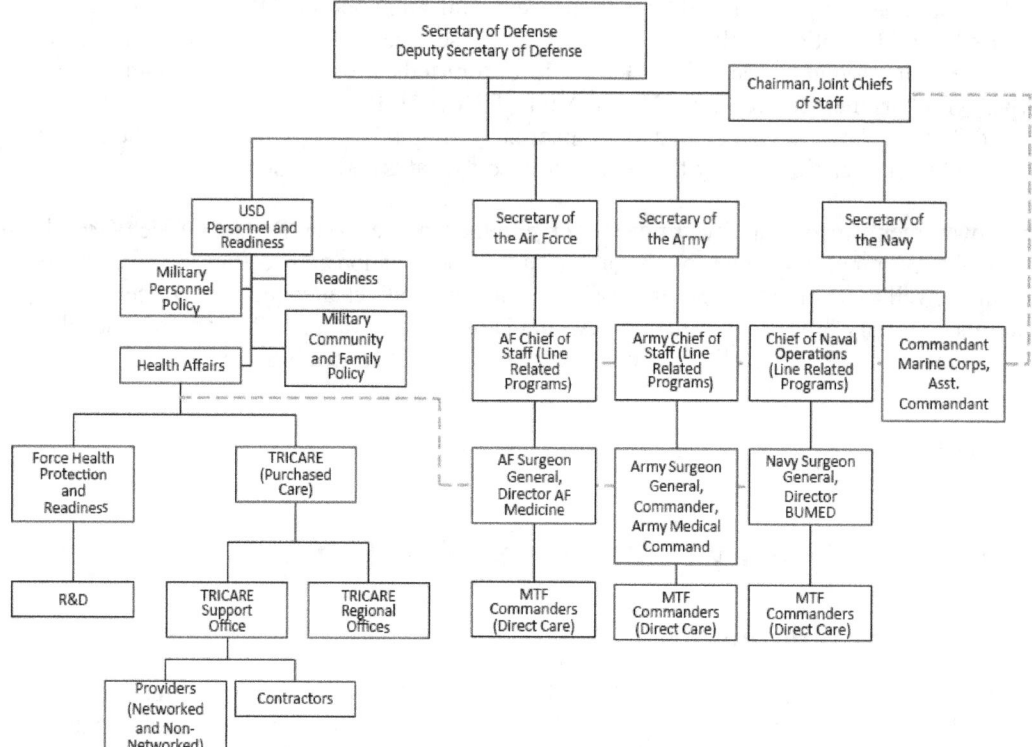

Source: Adapted from "Treatment for Post-Traumatic Stress Disorder in Military and Veteran Populations: Initial Assessment." Institute of Medicine. June 2012. Original information from Glover et al., 2011. "Continuum of care for post-traumatic stress in the US military enterprise." Proceedings of the 2011 Society of Health Systems Conference, Orlando, FL, February 17–19.

Notes: The Office of the Assistant Secretary of Defense for Health Affairs oversees Force Health Protection and Readiness programs and the purchased portion of TRICARE, and it has an administrative and policy relationship to the military treatment facilities (MTFs) (as indicated by the dotted line). BUMED = Bureau of Medicine and Surgery, R&D = Research and Development, USD = Undersecretary of Defense.

Within the services, the Surgeons General of the Army, Navy and Air Force retain considerable responsibility for managing military medical facilities and personnel. The Joint Staff Surgeon advises the Chairman of the Joint Chiefs of Staff.

The Surgeon General of the Army heads the U.S. Army Medical Command (MEDCOM) which along with the Office of the Surgeon General itself compose the Army Medical Department (AMEDD). The Surgeon General of the Army reports directly to the Secretary of the Army. MEDCOM commands fixed hospitals and other AMEDD commands and agencies. Field medical units, however, are under the command of the combat commanders.

The Surgeon General of the Navy reports to the Chief of Naval Operations through the Chief, Navy Staff and Vice Chief of Naval Operations and heads the Navy Bureau of Medicine and Surgery (BUMED), the headquarters command for Navy Medicine. All Defense Health Program resources allocated to the DON are administered by BUMED. Also within the Department of the Navy, the Medical Officer, U.S. Marine Corps advises the Commandant of the Marine Corps and Headquarters staff agencies on all matters about health services.

The Surgeon General of the Air Force serves as functional manager of the U.S. Air Force Medical Service, an element of Headquarters, U.S. Air Force. The Air Force Surgeon General advises the Secretary of the Air Force and Air Force Chief of Staff.

Potential Consolidation

The Final Report of the Task Force on Future of Military Health Care noted in 2007 that there has been considerable debate about the appropriate command and control structure for the military health system.[1] The current organizational structure has been observed by some to present an opportunity to gain efficiencies and save costs by consolidating administrative, management, and clinical functions. Alternatives to the current structure that have been suggested include a defense health agency or a unified medical command. Section 716 of the National Defense Authorization Act for Fiscal Year 2012 (P.L. 112-81) required the Secretary of Defense to submit to the congressional defense committees a report on military health system reorganization options. DOD's report, submitted March 2, 2012, considered 12 options and recommended Defense Health Agency with Service Military Treatment Facilities (MTFs) (similar to the current system) reporting that all of the Unified Medical Command options would increase costs.

Medical Personnel and Facilities

The military health system currently includes 56 hospitals and 365 clinics serving 9.7 million beneficiaries. It operates worldwide and employs some 58,369 civilians and 86,007 military personnel. Direct care costs include the provision of medical care directly to beneficiaries, the administrative requirements of a large medical establishment, and maintaining a capability to provide medical care to combat forces in case of hostilities. Civilian providers under contract to DOD have constituted a major portion of the defense health effort in recent years.

TRICARE Organization

The TRICARE Management Activity (TMA) listed above supervises and administers the TRICARE program. TMA is organized into six geographic health service regions:

- TRICARE North Region covering Connecticut, Delaware, the District of Columbia, Illinois, Indiana, Kentucky, Maine, Maryland, Massachusetts, Michigan, New Hampshire, New Jersey, New York, North Carolina, Ohio, Pennsylvania, Rhode Island, Vermont, Virginia, West Virginia, Wisconsin, and portions of Iowa, Missouri, and Tennessee. The TRICARE North regional contractor is currently Health Net Federal Services.

---

[1] Department of Defense, *Task Force on the Future of Military Health Care*, December 2007, pp. 113-116.

- TRICARE South Region covering Alabama, Arkansas, Florida, Georgia, Louisiana, Mississippi, Oklahoma, South Carolina, and most of Tennessee and Texas. The TRICARE South regional contractor is currently Humana Military Health Services.

- TRICARE West Region covering Alaska, Arizona, California, Colorado, Hawaii, Idaho, most of Iowa, Kansas, Minnesota, most of Missouri, Montana, Nebraska, Nevada, New Mexico, North Dakota, Oregon, South Dakota, portions of Texas, Utah, Washington, and Wyoming. The TRICARE West regional contractor is TriWest Healthcare Alliance.

- TRICARE Europe Area covering Europe, Africa, and the Middle East.

- TRICARE Latin America and Canada Area covering Central and South America, the Caribbean Basin, Canada, Puerto Rico and the Virgin Islands.

- TRICARE Pacific Area covering Guam, Japan, Korea, Asia, New Zealand, India and Western Pacific remote countries.

More information is available at http://www.TRICARE.mil/tma/AboutTMA.aspx.

2. What is the Unified Medical Budget?

ASD(HA) prepares and submits a unified medical budget which includes resources for the medical activities under his or her control within the DOD. The unified medical budget includes funding for all fixed medical treatment facilities/activities, including such costs as real property maintenance, environmental compliance, minor construction and base operations support. Funds for medical personnel and accrual payments to the Medicare Eligible Retiree Health Care Fund (MERHCF—see "3. What is the Medicare Eligible Retiree Health Care Fund (MERHCF)?," below) are also included. The unified medical budget does not include resources associated with combat support medical units/activities. In these instances the funding responsibility is assigned to military service combatant or support commands.

Unified medical budget funding has traditionally been appropriated in several places:

- The defense appropriations bill provides Operation and Maintenance (O&M), Procurement, and Research, Development, Test and Evaluation (RDT&E) funding under the heading "Defense Health Program."

- Funding for military medical personnel (doctors, corpsmen, and other health care providers) and TRICARE for Life accrual payments are generally provided in the defense appropriations bill under the "Military Personnel"(MILPERS) title.

- Funding for medical military construction (MILCON) is generally provided under the "Department of Defense" title of the military construction and veterans affairs bill.

- A standing authorization for transfers from the MERHCF to reimburse TRICARE for the cost of services provided to Medicare eligible retirees is provided by 10 U.S.C. 1113.

- Costs of war-related military health care are generally funded through supplemental appropriations bills.

Other resources are made available to the military health system from third-party collections authorized by 10 U.S.C. 1097b(b) and a number of other reimbursable program and transfer authorities. The President's budget typically refers to the unified medical budget request as its funding request for the military health system but only includes an exhibit for the DHP in the "Department of Defense - Military" chapter and exhibits for the MERHCF in the "Other Defense—Civil Programs" chapter of the Appendix volume. Medical MILCON and MILPERS request levels are generally found in DOD's budget submissions to Congress.

As illustrated in **Figure 2** below, the Obama Administration's FY2013 unified medical budget request[2] totals $48.7 billion and includes

- $32.5 billion for the Defense Health Program (not including "Wounded, Ill, and Injured" funding);
- $8.5 billion for military personnel;
- $1.0 billion for medical military construction; and
- $6.7 billion for accrual payments to the MERHCF.

Much more detailed breakouts are available in budget exhibits published by the Department of Defense at http://www.budget.mil.

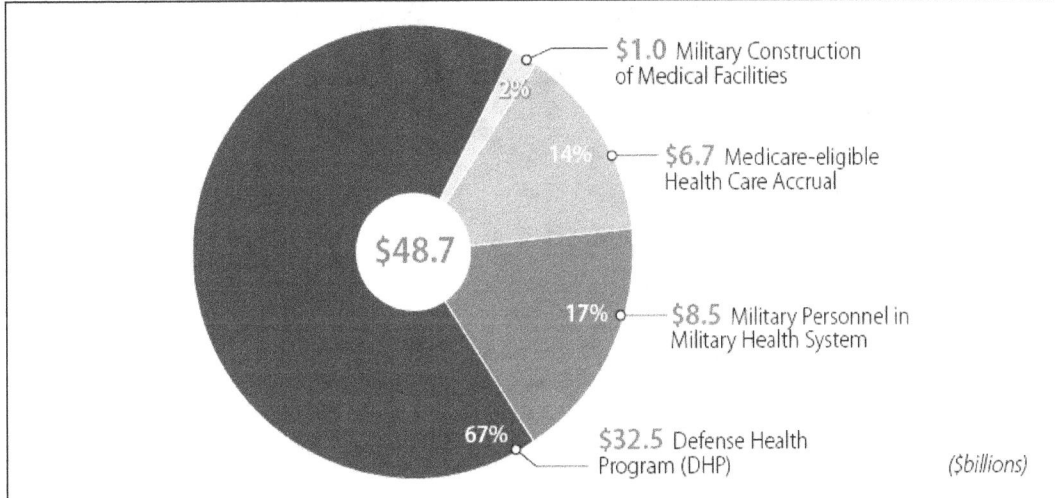

Figure 2. FY2013 Unified Medical Budget Request ($billions)

Source: Department of Defense FY2013 Budget Request Overview. Adapted by CRS Graphics.

---

[2] Department of Defense, *FY 2013 Budget Request Overview*, February 2012, pp. 5-2, Figure 5-1, http://comptroller.defense.gov/defbudget/fy2013/FY2013_Budget_Request_Overview_Book.pdf

3. What is the Medicare Eligible Retiree Health Care Fund (MERHCF)?

The Floyd D. Spence National Defense Authorization Act for Fiscal Year 2001(P.L. 106-398) directed the establishment of the Medicare-Eligible Retiree Health Care Fund to pay for Medicare-eligible retiree health care beginning on October 1, 2002, via a new program called TRICARE for Life. Prior to this date, care for Medicare-eligible beneficiaries was space-available care in MTFs. The MERHCF covers Medicare-eligible beneficiaries, regardless of age.

The FY2001 NDAA also established an independent three-member DOD Medicare-Eligible Retiree Health Care Board of Actuaries appointed by the Secretary of Defense. Accrual deposits into the Fund are made by the agencies who employ future beneficiaries (DOD and the other uniformed services including the Public Health Service, the Coast Guard, and the National Oceanic & Atmospheric Administration) based upon estimates of future TRICARE for Life expenses. Transfers out are made to the Defense Health Program based on estimates of the cost of care actually provided each year. As of September 30, 2011, the Fund had assets of over $163.6 billion to cover future expenses.[3]

The Board is required to review the actuarial status of the fund; to report annually to the Secretary of Defense, and to report to the President and Congress on the status of the fund at least every four years. The DOD Office of the Actuary provides all technical and administrative support to the Board. Within DOD, the Office of the Under Secretary of Defense for Personnel and Readiness, through the Office of the Assistant Secretary of Defense (OASD) for Health Affairs (HA) has as one of its missions operational oversight of the defense health program including management of the MERHCF. The Defense Finance and Accounting Service provides accounting and investment services for the fund.

4. What is TRICARE?

The Dependents Medical Care Act of 1956[4] provided a statutory basis for dependents of active duty members, retirees, and dependents of retirees to seek care at MTFs. Prior to this time, authority for such care was fragmented. The 1956 Act allowed DOD to contract for a health insurance plan for coverage of civilian hospital services for active duty dependents. Due to growing use of MTFs by eligible civilians and resource constraints, Congress adopted the Military Medical Benefits Amendments in 1966[5], which allowed DOD to contract with civilian health providers to provide non-hospital-based care to eligible dependents and retirees. Since 1966, civilian care to millions of dependents and retirees (and retirees' dependents) has been provided through a program still known in law as the Civilian Health and Medical Program of the Uniformed Services (CHAMPUS), but since 1994 more commonly known as TRICARE.

TRICARE has four main benefit plans: a health maintenance organization option (TRICARE Prime), a preferred provider option (TRICARE Extra), a fee-for-service option (TRICARE

---

[3] Department of Defense, *Fiscal Year 2011 Medicare-Eligible Retiree Health Care Fun Audited Financial Statements*, November 7, 2011, p. 5, http://comptroller.defense.gov/cfs/fy2011/12_Medicare_Eligible_Retiree_Health_Care_Fund/Fiscal_Year_2011_Medicare_Eligible_Retiree_Health_Care_Fund_Financial_Statements_and_Notes.pdf.

[4] P.L. 84-569.

[5] P.L 89-614.

Standard), and a Medicare wrap-around option (TRICARE for Life) for Medicare-eligible retirees. Other TRICARE plans include TRICARE Young Adult, TRICARE Reserve Select and TRICARE Retired Reserve. These plans are described below. TRICARE also includes a Pharmacy program and optional dental plans. Options available to beneficiaries vary by the beneficiary's relationship to a sponsor, sponsor's duty status, and location.

5. What are the Different TRICARE Plans?

TRICARE Prime

TRICARE Prime is a managed care option similar to a health maintenance organization—like such civilian arrangements, the plan's features include a primary care manager (either a military or a civilian health care provider) who oversees care and provides referrals to specialists. Referrals generally are required for such visits. To participate, beneficiaries must enroll and pay an annual enrollment fee, which is similar to an annual premium. Eligible beneficiaries may choose to enroll at any time. Enrollees receive first priority for appointments at military health care facilities and pay less out of pocket than do beneficiaries who use the other TRICARE plans. TRICARE Prime does not have an annual deductible.

Active duty servicemembers are required to use TRICARE Prime. They and their family members, as well as surviving spouses (during the first three years), and surviving dependent children are exempt from the annual enrollment fee. Retired servicemembers, their families, surviving spouses (after the first three years), eligible former spouses, and others are required to pay an annual enrollment fee, which is applied to the annual catastrophic out-of-pocket-limit .TRICARE Prime annual enrollment fees for military retirees were increased in FY2012 for new enrollees for the first time since the program began. Moving forward, under 10 U.S.C. 1097(e) TRICARE Prime enrollment fees will be subject to increases each fiscal year based on the annual retirement pay cost-of-living adjustment for the calendar year. For FY2013 (October 1, 2012– September 30, 2013) this enrollment fee is $269.28 for an individual and $538.56 for individual plus family coverage.

TRICARE Standard

TRICARE Standard is a traditional fee-for-service (FFS) option that does not require beneficiaries to enroll in order to participate. TRICARE Standard plan allows participants to use authorized out-of-network civilian providers, but it also requires users to pay higher out-of-pocket costs, generally 25% of the allowable charge for retirees and 20% for active duty family members. TRICARE Standard requires an annual deductible of $150/individual or $300/family for family members of sponsors at E-5 & above and $50/$100 for E-4 & below. Beneficiaries who use the Standard option must pay any difference between a provider's billed charges and the rate of reimbursement allowed under the plan.

TRICARE Extra

TRICARE Extra is also available to TRICARE Standard beneficiaries. It also has no formal enrollment requirement and mirrors a civilian preferred provider network. Network providers agree to accept a reduced payment from TRICARE and to file all claims for participants. By using network providers under TRICARE Extra, beneficiaries reduce their copayments, in general, to 20% of the allowable charge for retirees and 15% for active duty family members.

TRICARE Reserve Select

The TRICARE Reserve Select program was authorized by Section 701 of the Ronald W. Reagan National Defense Authorization Act for Fiscal Year 2005 (P.L. 108-375) which enacted Section 1076d of Title 10, United States Code. TRICARE Reserve Select is a premium-based health plan available worldwide for qualified Selected Reserve members of the Ready Reserve and their families. Servicemembers are not eligible for TRICARE Reserve Select if they are on active duty orders, covered under the Transitional Assistance Management Program, or eligible for or enrolled in the Federal Employees Health Benefits Program (FEHBP) or currently covered under the FEHBP through a family member. TRICARE Reserve Select provides benefits similar to TRICARE Standard. The government subsidizes the cost of the program with members paying 28% of the cost of the program in the form of premiums. For calendar year 2012, TRICARE Reserve Select premiums are $54.35 per month for member only coverage, and $192.89 per month for member and family coverage. For calendar year 2013, premiums are $51.62 per month for member only coverage, and $195.81 per month for member and family coverage.

TRICARE Retired Reserve

Section 705 of the National Defense Authorization Act for Fiscal Year 2010 (P.L. 111-84) added a new Section 1076e to Title 10, United States Code, to authorize a TRICARE coverage option for so-called "gray area" reservists, those who have retired but are too young to draw retirement pay. The program established under this authority is known as TRICARE Retired Reserve. Previously, such individuals were not eligible for any TRICARE coverage. This is a premium-based health plan that qualified retired members of the National Guard and Reserve under the age of 60 may purchase for themselves and eligible family members. It is similar to TRICARE Reserve Select, but differs in that there is no government subsidy as there is with TRICARE Reserve Select. As such, retired Reserve Component members who elect to purchase TRICARE Retired Reserve must pay the full cost of the calculated premium plus an additional administrative fee. Retired Reserve Component personnel who elect to participate in TRICARE Retired Reserve become eligible for the same TRICARE Standard, TRICARE Extra or TRICARE Prime options as active component retirees when the servicemember reaches age 60. Calendar year 2012 premiums for member only coverage are $419.72 per month and member-and-family premiums are $1,024.43 per month. Calendar year 2013 premiums for member only coverage are $402.11 per month and member-and-family premiums are $969.10 per month.

TRICARE Young Adult

Section 702 of the Ike Skelton National Defense Authorization Act for Fiscal Year 2011 (P.L. 111-383) amended Title 10, United States Code, to add a new Section 1110b, allowing unmarried children up to age 26, who are not otherwise eligible to enroll in an employer-sponsored plan, to purchase TRICARE coverage. The option established under this authority is known as "The TRICARE Young Adult Program." Unlike insurance coverage mandated by the Patient Protection and Affordable Care Act (P.L. 111-148) the TRICARE Young Adult Program provides individual coverage, rather than coverage under a family plan. A separate premium is charged. The law requires payment of a premium equal to the cost of the coverage as determined by the Secretary of Defense on an appropriate actuarial basis. For calendar year 2012 the monthly premium for a

TRICARE Young Adult (TYA) Prime enrollment is $201 and $176 for a TYA Standard enrollment.

TRICARE for Life

TRICARE for Life was created as "wrap-around" coverage to Medicare-eligible military retirees by Section 712 of the Floyd D. Spence National Defense Authorization Act for Fiscal Year 2001 (P.L. 106-398). TRICARE for Life functions as a second payer to Medicare, paying out-of-pocket costs for medical services covered under Medicare for beneficiaries who are entitled to Medicare Part A based on age, disability, or end-stage renal disease (ESRD). The beneficiaries are also eligible for medical benefits covered by TRICARE but not by Medicare. Prior to creation of the TRICARE for Life program, coverage for Medicare-eligible individuals was limited to space available care in military treatment facilities. In recognition of the requirement to enroll in Medicare Part B, TRICARE for Life cost-sharing with beneficiaries is limited and there is no enrollment charge.

In order to participate in TRICARE for Life, these TRICARE-eligible beneficiaries must enroll in and pay monthly premiums for Medicare Part B. TRICARE-eligible beneficiaries who are entitled to Medicare Part A based on age, disability, or ESRD, but decline Part B, lose eligibility for TRICARE benefits.[6] In addition, individuals who choose not to enroll in Medicare Part B upon becoming eligible may elect to do so later during an annual enrollment period; however, the Medicare Part B late enrollment penalty would apply.

6. How Much Does Military Health Care Cost Beneficiaries?

Active duty servicemembers receive medical care at no cost. Other beneficiaries pay differing amounts depending on their status, the TRICARE option enrolled in, and where they receive care. The tables below illustrate the costs to beneficiaries.

Table 1. Selected TRICARE Fees for Active Duty Personnel, Eligible Reservists, and Dependents

	Prime	Extra & Standard	
Annual Deductible	None	$150/individual or $300/family for E-5 and above; $50/ individual or $100/family below E-5	
Annual Enrollment Fee	None	None	
Annual Out-of-Pocket Limit	$1,000/family per fiscal year	$1,000/family per fiscal year	
Fees for Medical Services		in-network (TRICARE Extra)	out of network (TRICARE Standard)
Civilian Outpatient Visit	None	15% of negotiated rate	20% of allowable charge

---

[6] 10 U.S.C. §1086(d).

Military Medical Care: Questions and Answers

	Prime	Extra & Standard	
Emergency Room Visit	None	15% of negotiated rate	20% of allowable charge
Hospitalization	None	Greater of $25 per admission or $17.05/day.	Greater of $25 per admission or $17.05/day.
Civilian Inpatient Behavioral Health	None	Greater of $25 or $20/day.	Greater of $25 or $20/day.

Source: TRICARE website. Beneficiary costs current as of October 1, 2012.

For out-of-pocket limits, please see http://www.tricare.mil/mybenefit/home/Costs/HealthPlanCosts

For full beneficiary cost tables for TRICARE Standard and Extra, please see http://www.tricare.mil/mybenefit/home/Costs/HealthPlanCosts/TRICAREStandardExtra?

Table 2. Selected TRICARE Fees for Retirees Under Age 65 and Their Dependents

	Prime	Extra & Standard	
Annual Deductible	None	$150/individual or $300/family	
Annual Enrollment Fee	$269.28/individual or $538.56/family	None	
Annual Out-of-Pocket Limit	$3,000/family per fiscal year	$3,000/family per fiscal year	
Fees for Medical Services		in-network (TRICARE Extra)	out of network (TRICARE Standard)
Civilian Outpatient Visit	$12/visit	20% of negotiated rate	25% of allowable charge
Emergency Room Visit	$30/visit	20% of negotiated rate	25% of allowable charge
Hospitalization	Greater of $11/day or $25	Lesser of $250/day or 25% of billed charges for institutional services, plus 20% of separately billed services	Lesser of $708/day or 25% of billed charges for institutional services, plus 25% of separately billed services
Civilian Inpatient Behavioral Health	$40/day, no charge for separately billed professional services	20% of total charge plus 20% of allowable charge for separately billed professional services	High-Volume Hospital: 25% of hospital-specific per diem Low-Volume Hospital: Lesser of $208 per day or 25% of billed charges

Source: TRICARE website. Beneficiary costs current as of October 1, 2012.

For out-of-pocket limits, please see http://www.tricare.mil/mybenefit/home/Costs/HealthPlanCosts

For full beneficiary cost tables for TRICARE Prime for non-active duty families, please see http://www.tricare.mil/mybenefit/home/Costs/HealthPlanCosts/TRICAREPrimeOptions/EnrollmentFees? and http://www.tricare.mil/mybenefit/home/Costs/HealthPlanCosts/TRICAREPrimeOptions/NetworkCopayments?

For full beneficiary cost tables for TRICARE Standard and Extra, please see http://www.tricare.mil/mybenefit/home/Costs/HealthPlanCosts/TRICAREStandardExtra?

Military Medical Care: Questions and Answers

Table 3. Selected TRICARE Fees for Reserve Select and TRICARE Retired Reserve

	Reserve Select		Retired Reserve	
Annual Deductible	$150/individual or $300/family for E-5 and above; $50/$100 under E-5.		$150/individual or $300/family.	
Monthly Premium	$54.35/individual or $192.89/family		$419.72/individual or $1,024.43/family	
Annual Out-of-Pocket Limit	$1,000/family per fiscal year		$3,000/family per fiscal year	
Fees for Medical Services	in-network	out of network	in-network	out of network
Civilian Outpatient Visit	15% of negotiated rate	20% of negotiated rate	20% of allowable charge	25% of allowable charge
Emergency Room Visit	15% of negotiated rate	20% of negotiated rate	20% of allowable charge	25% of allowable charge
Hospitalization	Greater of $17.05/day or $25	Greater of $17.05/day or $25	Lesser of $250/day or 25% of billed charges for institutional services, plus 20% of separately billed services	Lesser of $708/day or 25% of billed charges for institutional services, plus 25% of separately billed services
Civilian Inpatient Behavioral Health	Greater of $20/day or $25	Greater of $20/day or $25	20% of total charge plus 20% of allowable charge for separately billed professional services	High-Volume Hospital: 25% of hospital-specific per diem Low-Volume Hospital: Lesser of $208 per day or 25% of billed charges

Source: TRICARE website. Beneficiary costs current as of October 1, 2012.

For out-of-pocket limits, please see http://www.tricare.mil/mybenefit/home/Costs/HealthPlanCosts

For full beneficiary cost tables for TRICARE Reserve Select, please see http://www.tricare.mil/mybenefit/home/Costs/HealthPlanCosts/TRICAREReserveSelect?.

For full beneficiary cost tables for TRICARE Retired Reserve, please see http://www.tricare.mil/mybenefit/home/Costs/HealthPlanCosts/TRICARERetiredReserve?

Table 4. Selected TRICARE Fees for TRICARE Young Adult

	Prime	Standard		
		Children of Active Duty Servicemembers and Sponsors Using TRICARE Reserve Select	*All Others including Children of Sponsors Using TRICARE Retired Reserve*	
Annual Deductible	None	$150/individual or $300/family	$150/individual or $300/family	
Monthly Premium	$201	$176	$176	
Annual Out-of-Pocket Limit	$3,000/family per fiscal year	$3,000/family per fiscal year	$3,000/family per fiscal year	
Fees for Medical Services		in-network / out of network	in-network	out of network

Congressional Research Service

	Prime	Standard			
		Children of Active Duty Servicemembers and Sponsors Using TRICARE Reserve Select		All Others including Children of Sponsors Using TRICARE Retired Reserve	
Civilian Outpatient Visit	$12/visit	15% of negotiated rate	20% of allowable charge	20% of negotiated rate	25% of allowable charge
Emergency Room Visit	$30/visit	15% of negotiated rate	20% of allowable charge	20% of negotiated rate	25% of allowable charge
Hospitalization	Greater of $11/day or $25	Greater of $17.05/day or $25	Greater of $17.05/day or $25	Lesser of $250/day or 25% of billed charges for institutional services, plus 20% of separately billed services	Lesser of $708/day or 25% of billed charges for institutional services, plus 25% of separately billed services
Civilian Inpatient Behavioral Health	$40/day, no charge for separately billed professional services	Greater of $20/day or $25	Greater of $20/day or $25	20% of total charge plus 20% of allowable charge for separately billed professional services	High-Volume Hospital: 25% of hospital-specific per diem Low-Volume Hospital: Lesser of $208 per day or 25% of billed charges

Source: TRICARE website. Beneficiary costs current as of October 1, 2012.

For out-of-pocket limits, please see http://www.tricare.mil/mybenefit/home/Costs/HealthPlanCosts

For full beneficiary cost tables for TRICARE Young Adult Prime, please see http://www.tricare.mil/mybenefit/home/Costs/HealthPlanCosts/TRICAREYoungAdult/PrimeOption

For full beneficiary cost tables for TRICARE Young Adult Standard, please see http://www.tricare.mil/mybenefit/home/Costs/HealthPlanCosts/TRICAREYoungAdult/StandardOption?

Table 5. TRICARE for Life Fees and Payment Structure

Type of Medical Service	What Medicare Pays	What TRICARE for Life Pays	What Beneficiary Pays
If covered by TRICARE and Medicare	Medicare's authorized amount	Remainder	$0
If covered by Medicare but not TRICARE	Medicare's authorized amount	$0	Medicare deductible and cost-share
If covered by TRICARE but not Medicare	$0	TRICARE's authorized amount	TRICARE deductible and cost-share
If not covered by TRICARE or Medicare	$0	$0	Full amount

Source: TRICARE, "TRICARE Choices at a Glance," May 2012, http://www.humana-military.com/library/pdf/cost-summary.pdf

7. What Is the DOD Pharmacy Benefit?

Those with access to military treatment facilities and those who are enrolled in TRICARE Prime receive prescribed pharmaceuticals free of charge. In accordance with the provisions of the FY2001 Defense Authorization Act (P.L. 106-398), effective April 1, 2001, retirees have access to DOD's National Mail Order Pharmacy and retail pharmacies in addition to pharmacies in military treatment facilities. Beneficiaries who turned 65 prior to April 1, 2001, qualify for the benefit whether or not they purchased Medicare Part B; beneficiaries who attain the age of 65 on or after April 1, 2001, must be enrolled in Medicare Part B to receive the pharmacy benefit. (There are deductibles for use of non-network pharmacies and co-payments for pharmaceuticals received from the National Mail Order Pharmacy and from retail pharmacies.)

Military pharmacies do not necessarily carry every pharmaceutical available; thus, even some with access to military facilities must have certain prescriptions filled in civilian pharmacies; for these prescriptions beneficiaries can be reimbursed through TRICARE.

In October 1997, DOD implemented the National Mail Order Pharmacy (subsequently known as the TRICARE Mail Order Pharmacy) that allows beneficiaries to obtain some pharmaceuticals by mail with small handling charges. The mail order program is designed to fill long-term prescriptions to treat conditions such as high blood pressure, asthma, or diabetes; it does not include medications that require immediate attention such as some antibiotics. Prescriptions filled by the TRICARE Mail Order Pharmacy in FY2012 cost $0 for a 90-day supply of a generic medication, $9 for a 90-day supply of a brand-name formulary medication, and $25 for a 90-day supply of a non-formulary medication.[7]

In 2004 DOD, in response to guidance in the FY2000 Defense Authorization Act (P.L. 106-65, Section 701), established a uniform formulary to discourage use of expensive pharmaceuticals when others are medically appropriate. Regulations to this effect were published in the Federal Register on April 1, 2004 (vol. 69, pp. 17035-17052). Section 703 of the FY2008 National Defense Authorization (P.L. 110-181) made pharmaceuticals purchased by TRICARE beneficiaries through retail pharmacies subject to federal pricing schedules. Prescriptions filled by a retail network pharmacy in FY2012 cost $5 for a 30-day supply of a generic medication, $12 for a 30-day supply of a brand-name formulary medication, and $25 for a 30-day supply of a non-formulary medication.[8]

The Secretary of Defense is authorized to set and adjust copayment requirements for the pharmacy program under 10 U.S.C. 1074g.

8. Who Is Eligible to Receive Care?

Eligibility for TRICARE is determined by the uniformed services and reported to the Defense Enrollment Eligibility Reporting System (DEERS). All eligible beneficiaries must have their eligibility status recorded in DEERS.

---

[7] TRICARE Pharmacy Benefit Handbook, Figure 5.1, p. 22, http://www.tricare.mil/mybenefit/Download/Forms/Pharmacy_HBK.pdf

[8] TRICARE Pharmacy Benefit Handbook, Figure 5.1, p. 22, http://www.tricare.mil/mybenefit/Download/Forms/Pharmacy_HBK.pdf

TRICARE beneficiaries can be divided into two main categories: sponsors and dependents. Sponsors are usually active duty servicemembers, National Guard/Reserve members or retired servicemembers. "Sponsor" refers to the person who is serving or who has served on active duty or in the National Guard or Reserves. "Dependent" is defined at 10 U.S.C. 1072, and includes a variety of relationships, for example, spouses, children, and certain unremarried former spouses.

Figure 3 illustrates the major categories of eligible beneficiaries.

Figure 3. Military Health System Eligible Beneficiaries (millions)

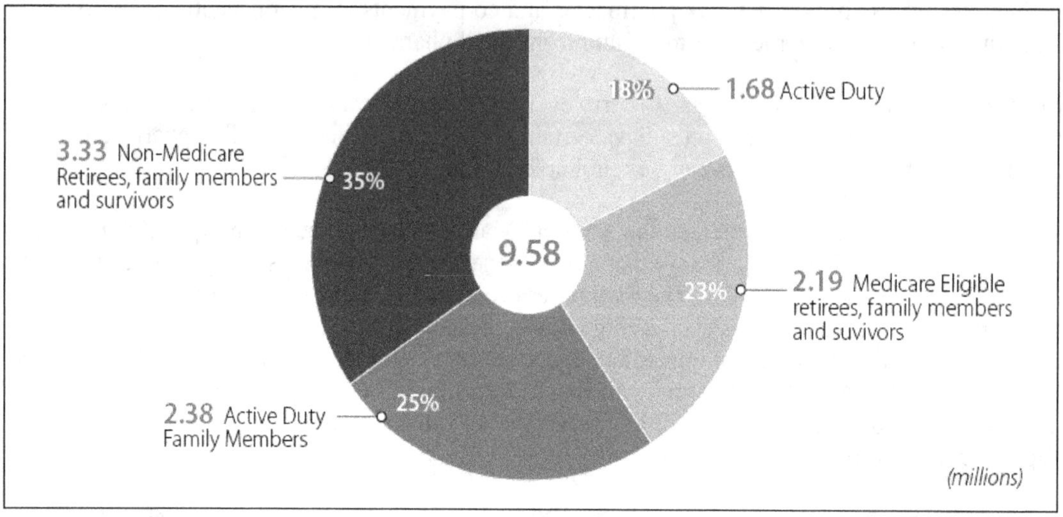

- 17% — 1.68 Active Duty
- 3.33 Non-Medicare Retirees, family members and survivors — 35%
- 2.19 Medicare Eligible retirees, family members and suvivors — 23%
- 2.38 Active Duty Family Members — 25%
- Total: 9.58 (millions)

Source: The President's Budget for FY2013, Appendix, "Department of Defense–Military Programs," p. 271. Adapted by CRS.

9. How Are Priorities for Care in Military Medical Facilities Assigned?

Active duty personnel, military retirees, and their respective dependents are not afforded equal access to care in military medical facilities. Active duty personnel receive top priority access and are "entitled" to health care in a military medical facility (10 U.S.C. 1074).

According to 10 U.S.C. 1076, dependents of active duty personnel are "entitled, upon request, to medical and dental care" on a space-available basis at a military medical facility. Title 10 U.S.C. 1074 states that "a member or former member of the uniformed services who *is* entitled to retired or retainer pay ... may, upon request, be given medical and dental care in any facility of the uniformed service" on a space-available basis.

This language entitles active duty dependents to medical and dental care subject to space-available limitations. No such entitlement or "right" is provided to retirees or their dependents. Instead, retirees and their dependents may be given medical and dental care, subject to the same space-available limitations. This language gives active duty personnel and their dependents priority in receiving medical and dental care at any facility of the uniformed services over military members entitled to receive retired pay and their dependents. The policy of providing active duty dependents priority over retirees in the receipt of medical and dental care in any facility of the uniformed services has existed in law since at least September 2, 1958 (P.L. 85-861).

Since the establishment of TRICARE and pursuant to the Defense Authorization Act of FY1996 (P.L. 104-106), DOD has established the following basic priorities (with certain special provisions):

> Priority 1: Active-duty servicemembers;
>
> Priority 2: Active-duty family members who are enrolled in TRICARE Prime;
>
> Priority 3: Retirees, their family members and survivors who are enrolled in TRICARE Prime;
>
> Priority 4: Active-duty family members who are not enrolled in TRICARE Prime;
>
> Priority 5: All other eligible persons.

The priority is given to active duty dependents to help them obtain care easily, and thus make it possible for active duty members to perform their military service without worrying about health care for their dependents. This is particularly important for active duty personnel who may be assigned overseas or aboard ship and separated from their dependents. As retirees are not subject to such imposed separations, they are considered to be in a better position to see that their dependents receive care, if care cannot be provided in a military facility. Thus, the role of health care delivery recognizes the unique needs of the military mission. The role of health care in the military is qualitatively different, and, therefore, not necessarily comparable to the civilian sector.

The benefits available to servicemembers or retirees, which require comparatively little or no contributions from the beneficiaries themselves, are considered by some to be a more generous benefit package than is available to civil servants or to most people in the private sector. Retirees may also be eligible to receive medical care at Department of Veterans Affairs (VA) medical facilities.[9]

10. What are the Long-Term Trends in Defense Health Costs?

Even as the number of active duty personnel in DOD declines over the next few years, costs associated with the military health system are expected to grow. Total military health system costs (excluding TRICARE for Life) increased between FY2009 and FY2011 for inpatient and outpatient services but declined for prescription drugs, due to the FY2008 NDAA requirement that the TRICARE retail pharmacy program be subject to the same pricing standards as other federal agencies.

DOD's FY2013 appropriations request for the Defense Health Program and the Medical Eligible Retiree Health Fund is approximately 7.4% of DOD's total FY2013 appropriations request.[10] The Congressional Budget Office (CBO) projects that the cost of the military health care system will

---

[9] See CRS Report RL32975, *Veterans' Medical Care: FY2006 Appropriations*, by Sidath Viranga Panangala.

[10] Comptroller, Department of Defense. National Defense Budget Estimates for FY2013, March 2012. Table 3-1, Reconciliation of Authorization, Appropriation, TOA and BA, by Program, by Appropriation. pp. 36-44, http://comptroller.defense.gov/defbudget/fy2013/FY13_Green_Book.pdf

grow from $51 billion in FY2013 (higher than DOD's FY2013 budget request of $47 billion) to $65 billion by FY2017 and $95 billion by FY2030.[11] Over the FYDP period from FY2013–FY2017, CBO's projection has average annual growth of 6.0%, compared with 2.6% in DOD's projection. Over the entire 2013–2030 period, CBO estimates the real (inflation-adjusted) growth rates in cost per user in the military health system would average 5.5% per year for pharmaceuticals, 4.7% for purchased care and contracts, and 3.3% for direct care and administration. Overall, DOD forecasts expect Defense Health Program costs to increase by 3.4% in FY2014, 3.35% in FY2015, 3.6% in FY2016 and 3.9% in FY2017, in constant FY2013 dollars.[12]

This cost growth stems in part from general inflation in the cost of health care, as well as an increasing percentage of care being provided to retirees and their dependents. DOD estimates that care provided to retirees and their dependents will make up over 65% of DOD health care costs by 2015, up from 43% in 1999.[13] A recent CBO analysis concludes that this increasing proportion of retirees participating in TRICARE is driven by "low out-of-pocket expenses for TRICARE beneficiaries (many of whose copayments, deductibles, and maximum annual out-of-pocket payments have remained unchanged or have decreased since the mid-1990s), combined with increased costs of alternative sources of health insurance coverage."[14] In addition, CBO found that TRICARE beneficiaries use both inpatient and outpatient care at rates significantly higher than people with other insurance, due to low out-of-pocket costs and other factors.

DOD proposed new fees and cost-sharing increases for retiree TRICARE plans in their FY2013 budget submission. The new fee proposals were generally based on recommendations by the 2007 Task Force on the Future of Military Health Care. This Congressionally-created Task Force found that, "because costs borne by retirees under age 65 have been fixed in dollar terms since 1996, when TRICARE was being established, the portion of medical care costs assumed by these military retirees has declined by a factor of 2-3."[15] Overall, "military health care premiums paid by individual military retirees under age 65 utilizing DOD's most popular plan (TRICARE Prime) have fallen from 11% to 4 %" of total health care costs.[16] These proposed cost-sharing increases and new fees would require new legislation.

---

[11] Congressional Budget Office, *Long Term Implications of the 2013 Future Years Defense Program*, p. 21, http://www.cbo.gov/sites/default/files/cbofiles/attachments/07-11-12-FYDP_forPosting_0.pdf.

[12] Comptroller, Department of Defense. *National Defense Budget Estimates for FY2013*, March 2012. Table 5-5, Department of Defense Deflators–TOA. p. 60, http://comptroller.defense.gov/defbudget/fy2013/FY13_Green_Book.pdf

[13] Department of Defense, Report of The Tenth Quadrennial Review of Military Compensation: Volume II Deferred and Noncash Compensation, July 2008, p. 45.

[14] Congressional Budget Office, *Long Term Implications of the 2013 Future Years Defense Program*, p. 21, http://www.cbo.gov/sites/default/files/cbofiles/attachments/07-11-12-FYDP_forPosting_0.pdf. p. 22.

[15] Department of Defense, subcommittee of the Defense Health Board, "Report of the Task Force on the Future of Military Health Care," December 2007, p. ES10, http://www.dcoe.health.mil/Content/Navigation/Documents/103-06-2-Home-Task_Force_FINAL_REPORT_122007.pdf

[16] Department of Defense, subcommittee of the Defense Health Board, "Report of the Task Force on the Future of Military Health Care," December 2007, p. 92, http://www.dcoe.health.mil/Content/Navigation/Documents/103-06-2-Home-Task_Force_FINAL_REPORT_122007.pdf

11. How Does the Patient Protection and Affordable Care Act Affect TRICARE?

In general, the Patient Protection and Affordable Care Act (PPACA)(P.L. 111-148) does not directly affect TRICARE administration, health care benefits, eligibility, or cost to beneficiaries.[17]

Section 3110 of the PPACA does open a special Medicare Part B enrollment window to enable certain individuals to gain coverage under the TRICARE for Life program.[18] The PPACA also waives the Medicare Part B late enrollment penalty during the 12-month special enrollment period (SEP) for military retirees, their spouses (including widows/widowers), and dependent children who are otherwise eligible for TRICARE and are entitled to Medicare Part A based on disability or end-stage renal disease, but have declined Part B. The Secretary of Defense is required to identify and notify individuals of their eligibility for the SEP; the Secretary of Health and Human Services (HHS) and the Commissioner for Social Security must support these efforts. Section 3110 of the PPACA was amended by the Medicare and Medicaid Extenders Act of 2010[19] to clarify that Section 3110 applies to Medicare Part B elections made on or after the date of enactment of the PPACA, which was on March 23, 2010.

12. How Are Private Health Care Providers Paid?

By law (P.L. 102-396) and Federal Regulation (32 CFR 199.14), health care providers treating TRICARE patients cannot bill for more than 115% of charges authorized by a DOD fee schedule. In some geographic areas, providers have been unwilling to accept TRICARE patients because of the limits on fees that can be charged. DOD has authority to grant exceptions. Statutes (10 U.S.C. 1079) also require that payment levels for health care services provided under TRICARE be aligned with Medicare's fee schedule "to the extent practicable." Over 90% of TRICARE payment levels are now equivalent to those authorized by Medicare, about 10% are higher, and steps are being taken to adjust some to Medicare levels.

For institutional providers of outpatient services, TRICARE recently published a final regulation[20] that became effective on May 1, 2009, implementing the TRICARE outpatient prospective payment system (OPPS). Under 10 U.S.C. 1079(h) and 1079(j)(2), DOD is required to use Medicare's reimbursement payment system for hospital outpatient services to the extent practicable. Under the OPPS, hospital outpatient services are paid on a rate-per-service basis that varies according to the Ambulatory Payment Classification (APC) group to which the services are assigned. Group services identified by Health Care Procedure Coding System (HCPCS) codes and descriptors within APC groups are the basis for setting payment rates under the hospital OPPS. To receive TRICARE reimbursement under the OPPS, providers must follow all Medicare specific coding requirements, except in those instances where the TRICARE Management Activity (TMA) develops specific APCs for those services that are unique to the TRICARE

---

[17] CRS Report R41198, *TRICARE and VA Health Care: Impact of the Patient Protection and Affordable Care Act (ACA)*, by Sidath Viranga Panangala and Don J. Jansen.

[18] §3110 of PPACA, P.L. 111-148.

[19] §201, P.L. 111-309.

[20] Department of Defense, "TRICARE: Outpatient Hospital Prospective Payment System (OPPS); Delay of Effective Date and Additional Opportunity for Public Comment," 74 *Federal Register* 6228, February 6, 2009.

beneficiary population. For inpatient services, TMA regularly publishes reimbursement schedules through the Federal Register.

13. What Is the Relationship of DOD Health Care to Medicare?

TRICARE and Medicare Payments to Providers and the Sustainable Growth Rate

Under 10 U.S.C. 1079, TRICARE is required to pay healthcare providers "to the extent practicable in accordance with the same reimbursement rules as apply to payments" under Medicare. This requirement was added by Section 731 of the National Defense Authorization Act for Fiscal Year 1996 (P.L. 104-106, February 10, 1996).

The Sustainable Growth Rate (SGR) is the statutory method for determining the annual updates to the Medicare physician fee schedule, created in the Budget Control Act of 1997 (see Section 1848 of the Social Security Act codified at 42 U.S.C. 1395w–4.) Under the SGR formula, if [Medicare] expenditures over a period are less than the cumulative spending target for the period, the annual update [to the provider fee schedule] is increased. However, if spending exceeds the cumulative spending target over a certain period, future updates are reduced to bring spending back in line with the target." In other words, if Medicare costs are greater than expected, the provider fees are reduced to bring overall Medicare expenditures down towards expected levels.

Each year since 2002, the sustainable growth rate (SGR) system, has produced a formula result (technically referred to as a "conversion factor") that would reduce reimbursement rates. With the exception of 2002, when a 4.8% decrease was applied, Congress has persistently declined to apply the SGR formula-driven reductions to provider fee rates through a series of temporary postponements known as "doc fixes."

Most recently, when President Obama signed the Middle Class Tax Relief and Job Creation Act of 2012 (P.L. 112-96) on February 22, 2012, the implementation of the SGR formula-driven reimbursement rates was again delayed until January 1, 2013. Absent legislation, the Medicare reimbursement rate reduction on January 1, 2013 has been estimated by the Department of Health and Human Services to be 27.4%.[21]

Although the law requires TRICARE reimbursement rates to be equal to Medicare rates "to the extent practicable," it does permit TRICARE to make exceptions to ensure an adequate network of providers or to eliminate a situation of severely impaired access to care.

Medicare and TRICARE for Life

Active duty military personnel have been fully covered by Social Security and have paid Social Security taxes since January 1, 1957. In 1965, Congress created Medicare under Title XVIII of

---

[21] Centers for Medicare and Medicaid Services, "Estimated Sustainable Growth Rate and Conversion Factor, for Medicare Payments to Physicians in 2012," Table 5, p. 7, http://www.cms.gov/Medicare/Medicare-Fee-for-Service-Payment/SustainableGRatesConFact/downloads/sgr2012f.pdf.

the Social Security Act to provide health insurance to people age 65 and older, regardless of income or medical history. Social Security coverage includes eligibility for health care coverage under Medicare at age 65.

In establishing CHAMPUS in 1966, it was the legislative intent of the Congress that retired members of the uniformed services and their eligible dependents be provided with medical care after they retire from the military, usually between their late-30s and mid-40s. However, Congress did not intend that CHAMPUS should replace Medicare as a supplemental benefit to military health care. For this reason, retirees became ineligible to receive CHAMPUS benefits when, at age 65, they become eligible for Medicare.

Many argued that the structure was inherently unfair because retirees lost TRICARE/CHAMPUS benefits at the stage in life when they were increasingly likely to need them. It was argued that military personnel had been promised free medical care for life, not just until age 65. After considerable debate over various options for ensuring medical care to retired beneficiaries, Congress in the FY2001 Defense Authorization Act (P.L. 106-259) provided that, beginning October 1, 2001, TRICARE pays out-of-pocket costs for services provided under Medicare for beneficiaries over age 64 if they are enrolled in Medicare Part B. This benefit is known as TRICARE for Life (TFL). Disabled persons under 65 who are entitled to Medicare may continue to receive CHAMPUS benefits as a second payer to Medicare Parts A and B (with some restrictions).

The requirement for enrollment in Medicare Part B, which had typical premiums of $99.40 per month in 2012[22], is a source of concern to some beneficiaries, especially those who did not enroll in Part B when they became 65 and thus must pay significant penalties. Some argue that this requirement is unfair since Part B enrollment was not originally a prerequisite for access to any DOD medical care. On the other hand, waiving the penalty for military retirees could be considered unfair to other Medicare-users who did not enroll in Part B upon turning 65. The Medicare Prescription Drug, Improvement, and Modernization Act (P.L. 108-173), passed in December 2003, waived penalties for military retirees in certain circumstances during an open season in 2004.[23]

14. What Medical Benefits are Available to Reservists?

Reservists and National Guardsmen (members of the "Reserve Component") who are serving on active duty have the same medical benefits as regular military personnel. Reserve personnel while on active duty for training and during weekly or monthly drills also are covered for illnesses incurred while on training or traveling to or from their duty station. In recent years, especially as members of the Reserve Component have had a larger role in combat operations overseas, Congress has broadened the medical benefits for Reservists. Those who have been notified that they are to be activated are now covered by TRICARE up to 90 days before reporting. Reservists who have served more than 30 days after having been called up for active duty in a contingency are eligible for 180 days of TRICARE coverage after the end of their service under the Transitional Assistance Management Program (TAMP). In addition, in 2004 Congress authorized

---

[22] Department of Health and Human Services, "Medicare Part B premiums for 2012 lower than projected," press release, 2011, http://www.hhs.gov/news/press/2011pres/10/20111027a.html.

[23] See out-of-print CRS Report RS21731, *Medicare: Part B Premium Penalty*, by Jennifer O'Sullivan, available upon request.

(in P.L. 108-375, Section 701) the TRICARE Reserve Select (TRS) program for Reserve Component members called to active duty, under Title 10, in support of a contingency operation after September 11, 2001. To be eligible for TRS, reservists must agree to stay in the Reserves for one or more years and must pay monthly premiums (in 2012, $54.35 for individual coverage, $192.89 for member and family coverage).

15. Have Military Personnel Been Promised Free Medical Care for Life?

Some military personnel and former military personnel maintain that they and their dependents were promised "free medical care for life" at the time of their enlistment. Such promises may have been made by military recruiters and in recruiting brochures; however, if they were made, they were not based upon laws or official regulations, which provide only for access to military medical facilities for non-active-duty personnel if space is available as described above. Space was not always available and TRICARE options could involve significant costs to beneficiaries. Rear Admiral Harold M. Koenig, the Deputy Assistant Secretary of Defense for Health Affairs, testified in May 1993: "We have a medical care program for life for our beneficiaries, and it is pretty well defined in the law. That easily gets interpreted to, or reinterpreted into, free medical care for the rest of your life. That is a pretty easy transition for people to make in their thinking, and it is pervasive. We [DOD] spend an incredible amount of effort trying to re-educate people [that] that is not their benefit."[24]

Dr. Stephen C. Joseph, Assistant Secretary of Defense for Health Affairs in April 1998, however, argued that because retirees believe they have had a promise of free care, the government did have an obligation. Joseph did not specify the precise extent of the obligation. The FY1998 Defense Authorization Act (P.L. 105-85) included (in Section 752) a finding that "many retired military personnel believe that they were promised lifetime health care in exchange for 20 or more years of service," and expressed the sense of Congress that "the United States has incurred a moral obligation to provide health care to members and [retired] members of the Armed Services." Further, it is necessary "to provide quality, affordable care to such retirees."

16. What is the Congressionally Directed Medical Research Program?

Many different entities within the Department of Defense request appropriations for and are funded to conduct a wide range of medical research. Over the last 17 years, Congress has supplemented the DOD appropriations to include additional unrequested funding for specific medical research funding. In 1992, Congress appropriated $25M for breast cancer research to be managed by DOD's U.S. Army Medical Research and Materiel Command (USAMRMC). The following year, Congress appropriated $210M to the DOD for extramural, peer-reviewed breast cancer research.

---

[24] U.S. Congress, House of Representatives, Committee on Armed Services, Military Forces and Personnel Subcommittee, 103rd Congress, 1st session, *National Defense Authorization Act for Fiscal Year 1994—H.R. 2401 and Oversight of Previously Authorized Programs*, Hearings, H.A.S.C. No. 103-13, April 27, 28, May 10, 11, and 13, 1993, p. 505.

Following this, DOD established the Congressionally Directed Medical Research Programs (CDMRP), within USAMRMC. The program now manages congressionally-directed appropriations totaling $6 billion through FY2010 for research on breast, prostate, and ovarian cancers; neurofibromatosis; military health; chronic myelogenous leukemia; tuberous sclerosis complex; autism; psychological health and traumatic brain injury; amyotrophic lateral sclerosis; Gulf War Illness; deployment-related health research; and other health concerns.[25] This additional, unrequested funding, now appears in the Defense Health Program RDT&E appropriation. Conference report language usually includes a table instructing the Department of Defense on how to allocate the additional funding to specific diseases and research areas. This guidance is not considered to be an earmark because the funding is used for peer-reviewed, competitively awarded research grants.

Table 6, below, depicts appropriations for selected CDMRP programs.

Table 6. Appropriation Levels by Fiscal Year(FY) for Selected CDMR Programs, FY2007–FY2012

(in millions of current dollars)

	FY 2007a	FY 2008b	FY 2009c	FY2010d	FY2011e	FY2012f
Amyotrophic Lateral Sclerosis	5	0	5	7.5	8	6.4
Autism	7.5	6.4	8	8	6.4	5.1
Bone Marrow Failure	0	0	5	3.75	4	3.2
Breast Cancer/Breast Cancer Research	127.5	138	150	150	150	120
Genetic Studies of Food Allergies	0	0	2.5	1.875	0	0
Gulf War Illness	0	10	8	8	8	10
Lung Cancer	0	0	20	15	12.8	10.2
Multiple Sclerosis	0	0	5	4.5	4.8	3.8
Neurofibromatosis	10	8	10	13.75	16	0
Ovarian Cancer	10	10	20	18.75	20	16
Peer-Reviewed Cancer	0	0	16	15	16	12.8
Peer-Reviewed Medical	0	0	50	50	50	50
Peer-Reviewed Orthopedic	0	0	51	22.5	24	30
Post-Traumatic Stress Disorder (PTSD)	151	0	0	0	0	0
Prostate Cancer	80	80	80	80	80	80
Psychological Health/Traumatic Brain Injury	150	0	165	120	100	135.5

---

[25] Department of Defense, *Congressionally Directed Medical Research Program: FY 2008 Annual Report*, September 30, 2008, pp. 1-2, http://cdmrp.army.mil/annreports/2008annrep/default.htm.

	FY 2007a	FY 2008b	FY 2009c	FY2010d	FY2011e	FY2012f
Spinal Cord Injury	0	0	35	11.25	12	9.6
Tuberous Sclerosis	0	4	6	6	6.4	5.1

Source: Congressionally Directed Medical Research Program, Annual Reports FY2007–FY2012, Recommendations accompanying the Defense Appropriations Acts.

Notes:

a. Funds appropriated by P.L. 110-5 (see H.Rept. 109-676 to H.R. 5631, September 25, 2006, pages 248-250), http://www.gpo.gov/fdsys/pkg/CRPT-109hrpt676/pdf/CRPT-109hrpt676.pdf

b. Funds appropriated by P.L. 110-116. See *Congressional Record*, November 6, 2007, p. H13119.

c. Funds appropriated by Division C of P.L. 110-329. See *Congressional Record*, September 24, 2008, pp. H9725–H9726.

d. Funds appropriated by P.L. 111-117. See *Congressional Record*, December 16, 2009, p. H15319–H15320, http://www.gpo.gov/fdsys/pkg/CREC-2009-12-16/pdf/CREC-2009-12-16-pt1-PgH15007-2.pdf#page=314

e. Funds appropriated by P.L. 112-10. See House Rules Committee' tables accompanying H.R. 1473, pp. 53-54, http://rules.house.gov/Media/file/FY11-Defense-Department-Base-tables.pdf

f. Funds appropriated by P.L. 112-74 (H.R. 2055). See House Rules Committee's tables accompanying H.R. 2055, 92A, p. 282, http://rules.house.gov/Media/file/PDF_112_1/legislativetext/H.R.2055crSOM/psConference%20Div%20A%20-%20SOM%20OCR.pdf

The CDMRP website (http://cdmrp.army.mil/) also provides specific descriptions and funding histories of the different research programs.

17. Other Frequently Asked Questions

Does TRICARE Cover Abortion?

10 U.S.C. 1093 provides that "Funds available to the Department of Defense may not be used to perform abortions except where the life of the mother would be endangered if the fetus were carried to term."

Does DOD Use Animals in Medical Research or Training?

Yes. DOD policy is that live animals will not be used for training and education except where, after exhaustive analysis, no alternatives are available. Currently approved uses include pre-deployment training for medical personnel and include infant intubation (ferrets); microsurgery (rodents); and combat trauma training (goats and swine).

Author Contact Information

Don J. Jansen
Analyst in Defense Health Care Policy
djansen@crs.loc.gov, 7-4769

Katherine Blakeley
Analyst in Foreign Affairs
kblakeley@crs.loc.gov, 7-7314

www.ingramcontent.com/pod-product-compliance
Lightning Source LLC
Chambersburg PA
CBHW081247180526
45171CB00005B/567